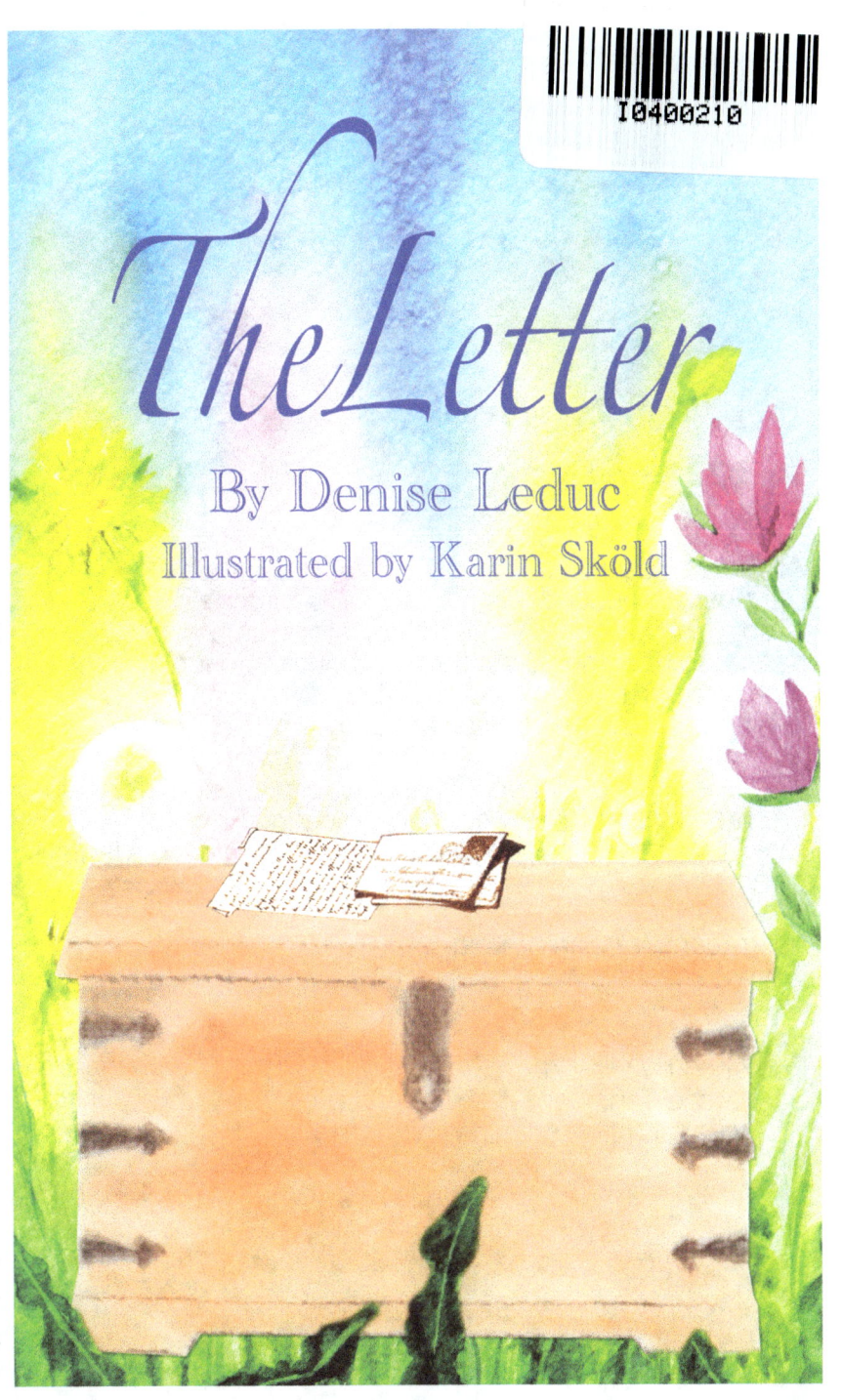

The Letter

By Denise Leduc
Illustrated by Karin Sköld

The Letter by Denise Leduc

© 2022 Denise Leduc
ISBN: 978-1-7782869-2-6

All Rights Reserved. No part of this publication may be reproduced, distributed, or transmitted in any form or by any means, or stored in a database or retrieval system, without the prior written permission of the publisher, except as permitted under the Canadian Copyright Act.

This is a work of fiction. All people, places, and incidents are products of the authors imagination. Any resemblances to people, living or dead, or any incidents is coincidental.

Illustrations by Karin Sköld
www.karinskold.com

Published by Lilac Arch Press
Saskatchewan, Canada
www.lilacarchpress.com

Dedicated to Barb,
who is always
loving, kind, and generous
—DL

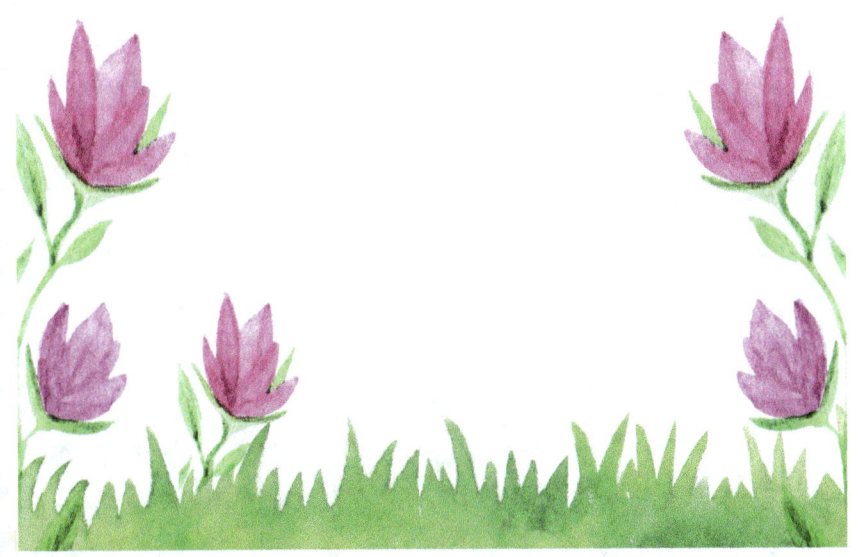

Table of Contents

Chapter 1–page 7

Chapter 2–page 15

Chapter 3–page 22

Chapter 4–page 27

Chapter 5–page 33

Chapter 6–page 39

Chapter 7–page 44

Chapter 8–page 53

Chapter 9–page 63

Chapter 10–page 68

Chapter 11–page 76

Chapter 12–page 81

Chapter 13–page 93

Chapter 14–page 100

Chapter 15–page 103

Chapter 16–page 110

Chapter 17–page 116

Afterword–page 118

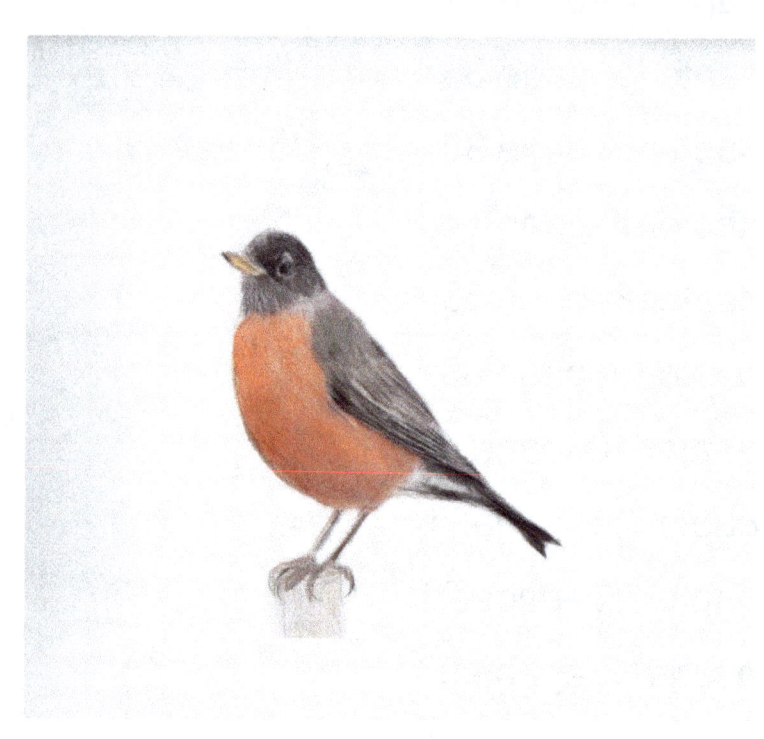

Chapter 1

Judy and Kate walked through the old red barn. It was the first warm day of spring. There had been a light rain earlier in the morning. Now, there was a freshness in the air. The robins were singing after a long winter, and one couldn't help but feel happy.

"This place is amazing," Judy said to her granddaughter.
"It sure is, Gram," Kate replied. "I can't believe all the beautiful stuff here."

The pair had taken a road trip to this rural antique shop in a barn. Kate had received a new job offer and was ready to move into her first apartment. She liked the vintage vibe and was hoping to find some treasures here.

Judy enjoyed browsing the space and seeing items that brought back memories of her youth

There were china teacups in the pattern her grandmother used to have. There were license plates of the style she remembered on her family's Buick. There was even a lamp that looked to be from the 1960s. This lamp looked like one Judy had in her first apartment with her roommate Janet.

Judy reached out and touched the smooth base of the lamp. She remembered the joy and fun she had found with Janet all those years ago as a young woman in the big city. She was happy for Kate and this new chapter of her life that she was about to begin.

A dark-haired woman greeted them. "Hi, I'm Emily. How can I help you folks today?"

Judy motioned to Kate.

"Just browsing," Kate answered. "I'm looking for some retro decor for my new place."

"You've come to the right spot," Emily said. "We've got lots in the barn, some stuff outside, and more buildings out back that are nice and full."

"Thank you," Kate smiled. Her attention was then drawn to a soft pink Victorian dress that she couldn't resist checking out.

Judy didn't need anything, but she wanted to buy something. So, slowly, she started to stroll through the barn, trying to take in all the charming items.

She paused at a large display of matchbox holders, the kind you didn't see in the stores anymore. She remembered always having one in the house while growing up. Here there were so many to choose from.

Kate reappeared by Judy's side. She was still looking through all the options and deciding which one to buy.

"Gram," she said, "You're where I left you. Did you have a chance to look around?"

"Not much," Judy confessed. "I found these matchbox holders and have been trying to decide which one to get. We used to have these when I was a kid."

Kate looked at them. "I don't think I've ever seen one," she admitted. Then, Kate added, "Well, take your time. We're not a hurry. We have the whole day, and I can do another tour around this place. There is so much stuff to see."

Eventually, Judy settled on a white matchbox holder with yellow daffodils. Yellow had been her mom's favorite color. She still missed her mom, who had passed away ten years ago, and thought of her often.

Judy thought she would remember her mom every time she saw the daffodils. That made her smile.

Finally, she started to make her way around some more displays. Every turn brought back a new memory.

After making her way to each building, she spotted Kate paying for her items.

"Hey Gram," Kate said. "I decided I had better pay for my stuff and stop adding to my pile, or I'm going to need a second job," she joked. "I will begin loading this stuff in my truck, but you take your time."

"I'm done," Judy said, showing Kate the matchbox holder.

"Oh, that's lovely," Kate said.

Judy got in line to pay. When it was her turn to approach the counter, she saw a wooden trunk on the other side. She didn't know why but knew she had to have it.

"Is that for sale?" she asked Emily as she pointed to the wooden trunk.

"Actually, yes, it is," Emily replied. "I got it in yesterday and haven't had a chance to put it out yet."

Judy surprised herself by saying, "I'll take it."

"Excellent. It's a great piece."

When Judy got to the vehicle, Kate had finished packing her treasures into her silver truck. Emily was behind Judy, carrying the wooden trunk.

"I hope you have room for one more thing," Judy said.

"Of course," Kate replied, "We can make it fit."

After they loaded the trunk in, the pair got into Kate's truck.

"I don't know what came over me," Judy confessed, "I saw the wooden trunk and had to have it. Before saying I would take it, I didn't even ask how much it was."

"Oh no," Kate said. "I hope it wasn't too much."

"No," Judy said. "It was a bargain. I'm not sure what I will do with it, though."

"I am sure we can think of something," Kate said. "Do you still want to go for ice cream?"

"Oh definitely," Judy smiled.

Chapter 1 Discussion Questions

1. What are your favorite parts of spring?
   _____
   _____

2. What are some things you remember from when you were young that could be in an antique shop today?
   _____
   _____

3. Who is a friend you remember from when you were younger?
   _____
   _____

4. What is the favorite color of someone you love?
   _____
   _____

5. What is your favorite kind of ice cream?
   _____

Chapter 2

After their ice cream, Judy and Kate stopped at some garden centers along their route home. It was late afternoon when they finally arrived back at Judy's house.

"I will grab the wooden trunk," Kate offered as they hopped out of her truck.

As she took it into Judy's home, she remarked, "It is charming. I have to get a picture of it."

She set it down, and they looked over it more. It wasn't very big, just over two feet long and one foot wide. The wood was a light honey color. It was smooth in some areas. Yet, other areas were quite worn and rough. The latches were leather. The inside was lined with an old beige floral paper.

"What do you think you might do with it, Gram," Kate asked.

"I don't know yet. I suppose I could store my knitting in it. Or it would be a good place for some old keepsakes."

"I can come over next weekend and do a light sanding on the rougher wood," Kate offered.

"That would be nice. I can clean it up before that," Judy said. "I will give it a good wash and take that old floral paper out."

"We could go to the fabric store and get something new to line it with," Kate offered.

"That sounds fun," Judy agreed. "I love going to the fabric store and seeing all the pretty options."

"Plaid is always a good choice," Kate grinned.

It was well known in the family that Kate was wild about plaid. She had plaid clothes, plaid shoes, and plaid purses.

She had lots of plaid blankets and even had some plaid furniture.

"I was thinking something a little plainer," Judy said, "Maybe something in a chocolate brown."

"Or something with a springtime theme," Kate suggested with a smile. "Tulips, robins' eggs, bunnies are all a nice choice."

They both laughed. Judy liked neutrals and simplicity, while Kate preferred vibrant, colorful, and fun.

Kate said goodbye to her grandma and left.

Alone Judy went over to the wooden trunk again. She still didn't know what had made her buy it, but she was glad.

She grabbed a bowl of soapy water and a cloth, then gently started to wash the outside of the wooden trunk. She liked the smell of the pine cleaner she was using. It made everything seem fresh.

After washing the outside, she opened the wooden trunk. Before cleaning the inside, she might as well take out that old floral paper. The paper had browned and had a light layer of dust. It had started to tear on its own. It was easy to peel it away from the trunk.

She had removed it from all the sides and was beginning to tear it away from the bottom. Then something underneath the paper caught her eye. Gently she pried a corner of the paper up.

Underneath was an old weathered envelope. Being extra careful, Judy lifted the envelope. She saw that it was addressed to Mrs. Alva Munro. She turned it over and saw it had been sealed and never opened.

She took the envelope over to her kitchen table and laid it down. She was curious. She had so many questions.

What was this letter doing in this wooden trunk underneath the paper? Who was Alva Munro? Why hadn't she received this letter? What did the letter say? Was it important?

Judy wanted to open the letter and read it, but she wasn't sure if she should. She touched the paper again. It seemed so delicate.

Judy put the letter in her china cabinet for safekeeping until she knew what to do with it.

Yet, all that evening, Judy couldn't stop thinking about the letter and what it might say. She stayed awake well past midnight wondering about the mysterious letter.

Chapter 2 Discussion Questions

1. What would you keep in the wooden chest?
   _____
   _____

2. What kind of fabric would be nice for the wooden chest?
   _____
   _____

3. What are some of your favorite scents?
   _____
   _____

4. What would you do if you found a mysterious letter?
   _____
   _____

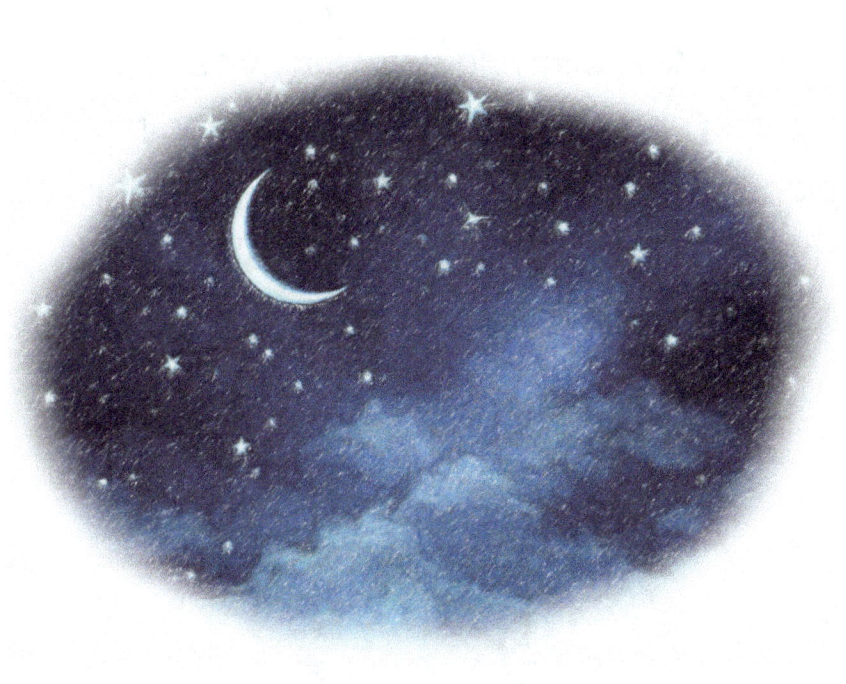

Chapter 3

Early the following day, Judy was still thinking about the letter. She watched her grandmother's old clock. Finally, when she knew Kate would be on a break she picked up the phone and called her.

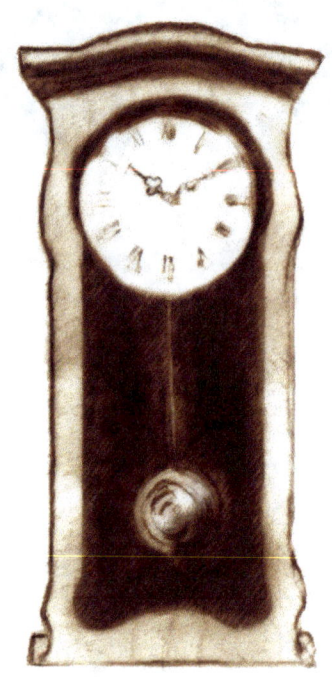

"Hello," Kate said.

"Hello dear," Judy replied. "I wanted to call and tell you that I found an old letter when I was washing out that wooden trunk."

"Well, that sounds interesting," said Kate. "Tell me more. What did it say?"

"I don't know," Judy admitted. "It was still sealed, and I can't decide if I should open it or not."

Judy told Kate how the letter was addressed to Mrs. Alva Munro. She shared that the address was in Fox Creek. She had also noticed the stamp on the envelope was from 1955.

"Wow, Gram," Kate said. "You did find a treasure."

As they chatted, Kate went on her computer to look up where Fox Creek was. She learned it was a three-hour drive west of the small town of Patterson where they lived.

An internet search showed that Fox Creek Is a tiny village. It had a population of approximately only 60 people.

"I imagine someone in Fox Creek might know Alva Munro or the Munro family," Kate suggested.

Kate did another internet search while she and Judy were still on the phone. This time she searched the name Alva Munro. There was an Alva Munro who was a nurse in Winnipeg. Surprisingly, there was a teenage girl with purple hair named Alva Munro. Yet, Kate could not find an Alva Munro from the Fox Creek area or an Alva Munro from around 1955.

"I don't know what to say, Gram. You could open the letter for some clues."

"I don't know," Judy paused to give it some more thought. "I don't know if opening someone else's mail is right, even if it was from that long ago."

"We could drive one weekend to Fox Creek and poke around. There might still be family in the area."

"Well, you know I always love to go for a country drive," Judy said, "but that is a bit of a way to travel. It might turn out to be a wild goose chase."

Suddenly, Judy had an idea.

"I know what I can do," she said. "I will go up to the library. The librarian, Terri, is full of information. She might be able to lead me in the right direction or give me some ideas."

"Terri is awesome," Kate agreed. "That's a great idea, Gram. Please keep me updated on what you learn. I'm very curious about your letter too."

"I knew I had to buy that wooden trunk," Judy said. "I feel I was meant to find this letter for some reason."

Chapter 3 Discussion Questions

1. How do you imagine a place named Fox Creek might be?
   _____
   _____

2. Do you like road trips and country drives?
   _____

3. What is an exciting place you have traveled to?
   _____
   _____

4. Judy and Kate seem to like their local library. Has there been a library that's been remarkable to you?
   _____
   _____
   _____

Chapter 4

After a poached egg and toast for a late breakfast, Judy got dressed and ready to go to the library. There was a light spring rain. Judy put on her raincoat and rubber boots and grabbed an umbrella.

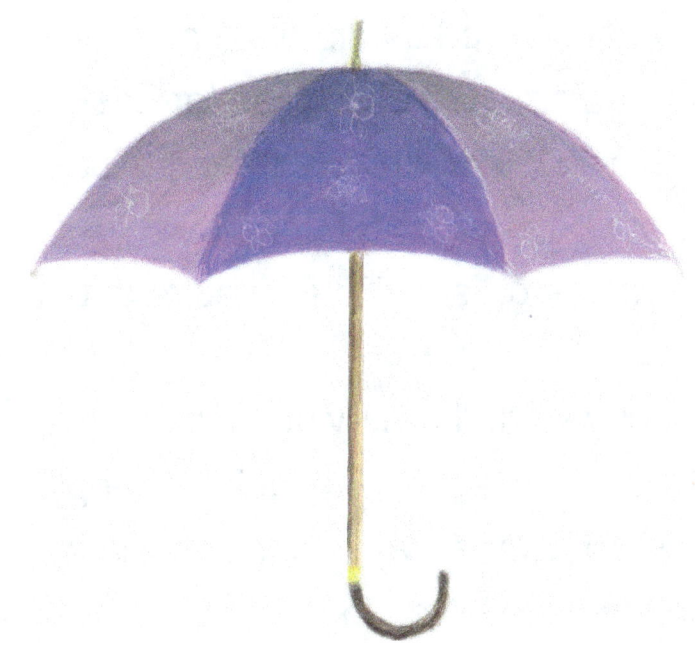

Walking the three blocks to the library, she noticed that the grass was beginning to turn green. In the neighbors' gardens, bulbs were already starting to add some color around town.

A fat squirrel scurried up a tree. The squirrel jumped from one branch to another. Finally, the squirrel looked down and seemed to scold Judy for disturbing her.

When Judy entered the library, she saw that the librarian, Terri, had decorated for Easter. There was also lots of artwork from the local children.

"Good morning," said Terri. "You're out on a rainy day."

" Yes," Judy said. "I am trying to find some information. Is there a way to look for people from the 1950s? Or a way to find information about the town they lived in?"

Judy then shared the details of finding the letter with Terri

"Well," Terri said, "We have some books about the small towns around this area. I'm not sure if it will give you all the details about folks from that far back, but it might give you some leads."

Terri took Judy over to a shelf; there were large books in alphabetical order for dozens of small towns. Right away Terri located the one for Fox Creek and pulled it down.

The pair opened the thick book at the table. They started scanning it, looking for anything that might stand out.

The book started with black and white photos of the town beginning in 1909. In that first photograph were several men standing in front of a wagon with some horses. In the background were a few wooden buildings.

Judy turned the page. On the second page was a photograph of a family with small children in front of a sod shack. Judy tried to imagine what it must have been like to raise children in such a home.

Judy skimmed over the following several pages that seemed to be more of the village of Fox Creek over the years. She wanted to look at them, but was more interested in information she might find about Alva Munro.

She noted that after the opening pages with pictures of the town, there was a section on family histories. Quickly, Judy flipped through the pages to the letter M.

She was thrilled to see there was indeed a section dedicated to the last name, Munro. She realized, though, that it was quite an extensive section.

"Would I be able to check this book out?" she asked Terri.

"Of course," Terri replied.

After Terri scanned the book through the computer system, she said, "You will have to let me know what you find out. This is an interesting puzzle you have stumbled upon."

The ladies said their goodbyes. As Judy stepped outside she saw the rain had cleared. The sky was blue, and the sun was shining. It was going to be a beautiful day.

Chapter 4 Discussion Questions

1. Would you go for a walk in the rain or wait for sunny weather?
   _____

2. What spring bulbs are your favorite?
   _____

3. Do you like looking at old photographs? What are your favorite types of things to see?
   _____
   _____

4. What is an old photograph that you remember?
   _____
   _____

Chapter 5

Judy wasn't sure why, but once she got home, she put the Fox Creek book on the table and went to do some chores. While she washed some dishes and swept up the floor, she was still thinking about the letter.

Judy took a lawn chair and matching side table out of her shed. She had not had this furniture out since the fall. She quickly wiped it down. Then she placed it underneath the old oak tree that was starting to show buds.

Going back inside the house, Judy made herself a cup of tea. Then, she placed some ginger snaps on a little plate. It was a good time for a little snack.

Judy's black and white cat, Frank Sinatra, came and brushed against her leg. He had seen her take out the milk for her tea. He meowed loudly, letting her know that he'd like some too

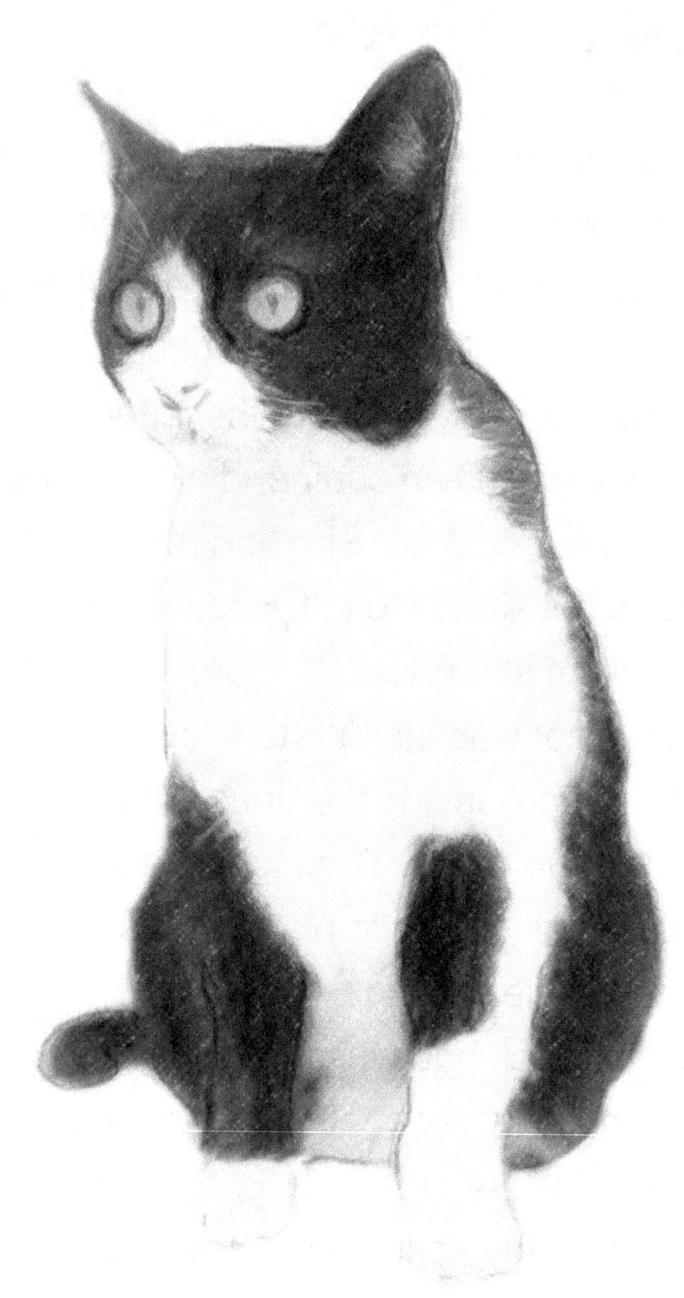

Judy loved him so much and could never resist his meows. She went over to his little red bowl and filled it with milk. He brushed against her again. This time he purred.

Judy took her snack outside. Then went back in and waited for Frank Sinatra to finish his milk. She knew he would want to join her outside. He enjoyed going out to lay on the grass to watch the birds. He never bothered them, and he never went far. He was a good companion.

Finally, he was ready. Judy grabbed the book and opened the door. Once outside, Frank Sinatra went beside the lawn chair and found a comfy spot for himself.

Judy decided to add some water to the bird bath and food to the bird feeder before sitting down. Then, she noticed robins building a nest in the lilac bushes. She looked forward to seeing the babies in a few weeks and watching them grow.

Judy also looked forward to the lilac blooms when they eventually arrived.

Judy settled into her chair with a sigh. She sipped her tea. She had one ginger snap. Then she rubbed her fingers over the book cover for the village of Fox Creek. She knew there was something interesting within these pages.

When she opened the book, she looked at the photographs on the front again. Again, she enjoyed seeing what the village of Fox Creek looked like over one hundred years ago.

There was a picture of the first church in town. There was a picture of the early railroad. There were several pictures of the main street. Seeing these pictures for the first time made Judy think of her own town of Patterson.

Judy had lived in Patterson so long that she no longer noticed all the details. Patterson was about as old as Fox Creek.

She made up her mind to make a point of really seeing the unique elements of her town on her future walks. She thought she should even visit the local museum sometime soon. It had been a long time since she had been there.

Judy looked through all the photographs at the front of the book, then turned to the family histories and the letter M.

Judy slowly turned the pages until she came to a page with bold letters spelled out, Munro.

Judy started looking carefully at all the photographs and the captions beneath them. Finally, on the seventh page about the family, she found what she was looking for, a photograph dated 1948. Smiling through the page and over the years was a beautiful blonde woman wearing a polka dot dress. Her hair was in victory rolls. In her arms was a toddler. The young woman looked lovingly at the child. The woman was Alva Munro.

Chapter 5 Discussion Questions

1. Have you had a pet that was special to you?
   _____

2. Do you have a favorite Frank Sinatra song?
   _____

3. What flowers do you get excited to see in the spring or summer?
   _____

4. What are your favorite birds?
   _____

5. Is there a hairstyle or fashion from your past that you fondly remember?
   _____

6. Is there a hairstyle or fashion from your past that you now think was silly?
   _____

Chapter 6

Outside Judy had her cat to one side and spring bulbs on the other. She read and reread the pages dedicated to the Munro family. She learned that the Munro family had been one of the first to settle Fox Creek. She realized that the family had been quite prosperous. Many of the Munro men had served in WWII. Some did not return home. One young Munro woman had been the local schoolteacher.

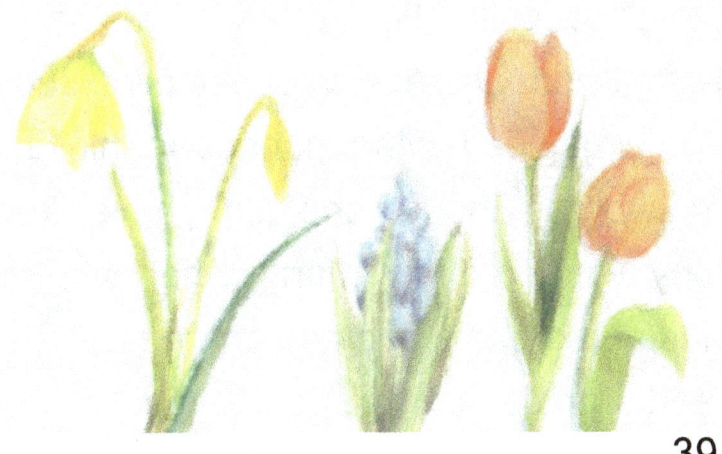

It was fascinating to learn about this family. It reminded her that everyone has a story.

Even I have a story, Judy thought. She started to think about things others might find interesting in her life. She had been the first girl in her family to go to college. In college, she had been front row to see the Beatles when they came to Toronto. She was even certain Paul had winked at her.

Before she had married, Judy had a brief stint as a stewardess. That was what you called them back in those days. She knew the job was now called flight attendant as her oldest granddaughter, Liz, was a pilot. Judy couldn't imagine having that opportunity as a young woman, though she might have liked it.

Judy wondered how many of her own stories and dreams she had shared with her kid and grandkids. She spent lots of time with Kate.

They always chatted, but she wasn't sure how many stories of her youth she had shared.

Judy thought she should write some of her stories down for her grandchildren. They knew her as Grandma or Gram. She wasn't sure if they ever thought of her being a child, a teenager, or a young woman.

A book of family photos with some of her stories might be a lovely keepsake.

After supper, Judy called Kate to share what she had learned about the Munro family.

"Well, that is interesting," Kate said. "Have you decided what to do with the letter yet?"

She still didn't know what she should do with the letter. The way she was raised, you never opened someone else's mail. Yet, she also realized that Alva Munro may not even be alive.

"No," Judy admitted.

Judy paused to consider more before adding, "I wish there was a way to get in touch with someone from Alva Munro's family. Then I could give it to them. That would make me happy."

"Well," Kate said, "I guess there is only one thing for us to do. We need to take a trip to Fox Creek next weekend."

Chapter 6 Questions

1. Judy realizes that everyone has a story. What is a story about you or your family? Have you shared your story with others?

   _____
   _____
   _____
   _____

2. What work have you done?

   _____

3. What work might you have liked to do but didn't have the opportunity?

   _____

4. Kate is a helpful granddaughter. Who is someone helpful in your life?

   _____

5. Is there a concert you have been to?

   _____

6. What Beatles songs do you like?

   _____

Chapter 7

On Saturday, Kate picked Judy up at 7 am. It was another warm spring day. They figured that with Fox Creek being three hours away, they had plenty of time to make it a leisurely day.

They had decided they would stop for breakfast on their way. They would also make stops along the journey whenever anything caught their interest.

Judy had brought the letter with her in case they lucked out. She wasn't sure what to expect when they got to Fox Creek. Were they just going to knock on doors in the village? She wasn't sure about this plan.

But, Kate seemed confident that it would all work. Judy had always loved going for drives. No matter what, she was sure they would have a fun time together.

"What should we listen to today, Gram?" Kate asked.

Kate always let Judy pick the music when they went on drives. She loved how Kate could pull up so much music all on her phone.

Judy remembered listening to the radio in the car with her family as a child. When she got her first car, an eight-track player was in it. When she had kids of her own, the cars played cassette tapes. Now, Kate had thousands of songs available on her phone. Technology was marvelous.

"Oh, I don't know," Judy said. There was so much to choose from she didn't know what to pick. "Surprise me."

Kate smirked, "Okay," she said.

She ended up putting on some Kenny Rogers. "Do you remember Grandpa putting this record on when we'd play euchre?" Kate asked Judy.

Judy smiled. She did remember. Her husband had taught all the grandkids to play euchre and bridge. He was a country music fan and would always put on music when playing cards. It had been fifteen years since he passed away, but his thoughts still made her smile. He had been a good man.

They listened for quite a while. When the song, "The Gambler", finally came on, Kate spotted a roadside diner.

"Should we stop here?" she asked.

"I could eat," Judy replied.

Inside, Kate ordered waffles with whipped cream and blueberries. Judy had classic bacon and eggs.

A little shop with the diner carried locally made goods. Kate learned the owners were also beekeepers. She was delighted to find their flavored honey.

Judy looked around. She found a cookbook for sale that supported the local fire hall. She loved getting new cookbooks and liked supporting a good cause.

After completing their purchases, they were back on the road. This time Kate put on Willie Nelson's, "On the Road Again".

By now, the sun was blazing. Fluffy, white clouds dotted the blue sky. They traveled miles in silence, enjoying the music and the spring day.

They came to an intersection, and Kate said, "I think this is our turn."

As they started in this new direction, it didn't take long for the landscape to change. After a few minutes, the pavement turned to gravel. They noticed more cows in the fields they passed by. Now and then, they saw an old farmhouse.

Kate slowed down as potholes started to get a little deeper and a little more frequent.

"This is like an obstacle course," she chuckled as she dodged yet another large pothole.

They drove a little further when Judy noted, "It is so quiet out here."

Kate looked around. "You're right," she said as she pulled the truck over to the side of the road.

The pair got out of the car to stretch their legs. Then, they went for a bit of a stroll before stopping.

"Listen," whispered Judy.

Kate smiled. There was not a sound. Around them, there was only stillness and silence.

"I don't see a living creature," Judy said. "Not a bird in the sky, not an insect, not a mouse on the ground."

Judy and Kate were slow and watchful on the walk back to the car. Each was looking for some sign of life in this place.

"You don't often experience such quiet," Judy mused.

Back in the car, they continued toward their destination. Judy watched the fields roll by. Soon grains would be starting to fill the landscape. She began to think about her garden and what plants she might grow this year.

"Oh, look," Kate pointed at a sign that showed they had to make another turn for Fox Creek. It said that Fox Creek was only 14 miles away.

Kate slowed down. As soon as they made the turn, they both gasped and together said, "Oh wow!"

Right in front of them were a mama moose and her baby. Kate slowed to a stop. She didn't want to frighten the giant animal. The mama moose was calm as she looked at them.

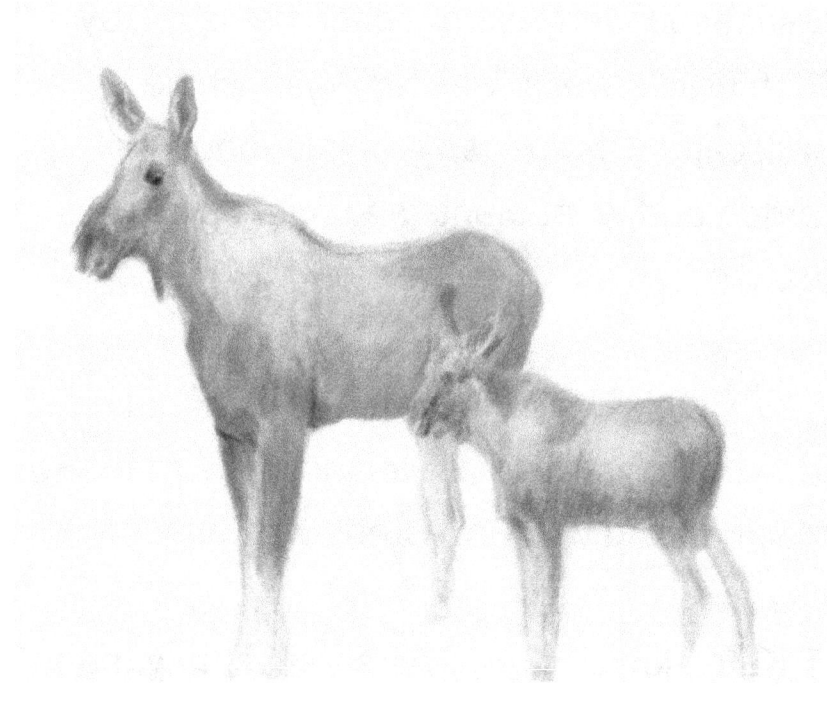

Judy and Kate had a chance to grab their cameras and snap some pictures. It was almost like the moose was posing for them. Then, after a few moments, the moose started to make her way to the other side of the road. Her baby followed.

"That was amazing," Kate exclaimed.
Judy agreed.

It didn't take long for them to go the rest of the distance to Fox Creek. On the right was a white sign. In bold letters, it said, Welcome to Fox Creek. From behind the W, a picture of a fox peeked out. The sign stated that the village had formed in 1909.

Judy took a deep breath. It has been a pleasant journey so far. She wasn't sure what to expect now that they were here.

Chapter 7 Discussion Questions

1. What is your favorite music?
   _____

2. Do you have memories of the radio, eight tracks, or cassette tapes?
   _____
   _____

3. What card games do you enjoy?
   _____
   _____

4. Have you had a garden?
   _____

5. Do you enjoy gardening?
   _____

6. What things have you liked to grow in a garden?
   _____

7. What animals do you like to see in the wild?
   _____

Chapter 8

They turned into the village of Fox Creek. A flag blew in the soft breeze. Beside the flag was a statue of a giant metal sunflower.

They continued down the street and saw a playground on the left. Three children were playing there while a teenager watched. One child was digging in the sand while another was swinging on a swing, and the third was trying to climb up the slide. Judy chuckled and shook her head.

Beside it was an old schoolhouse. It looked like it had been abandoned many years ago, but the sign was still there. Judy imagined what it must have been like. She imagined all the children coming to this one-room schoolhouse a century ago.

Kate must have been thinking the same because she asked, "Did you go to a one-room schoolhouse, Gram?"

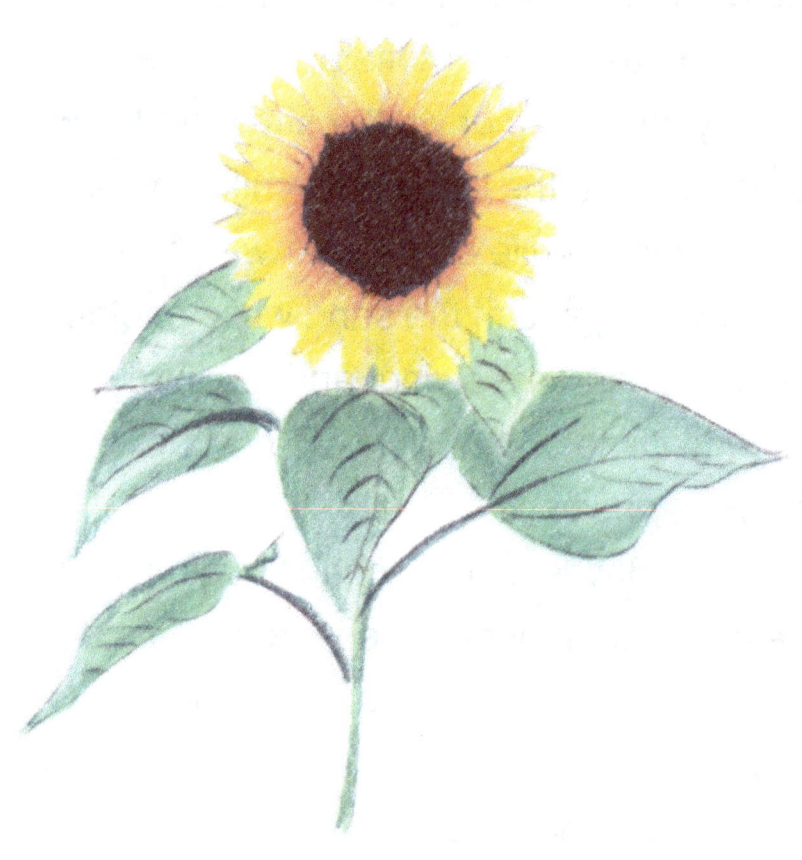

"How old do you think I am," Judy scoffed.

Kate shrugged.

"You might not believe it, but when I was a child, we even had electricity," Judy joked.

Kate laughed, "I didn't mean any offense. I didn't know how long schoolhouses like that would have been common in these small towns."

As they approached a crossroads, they came to a stop. Kate looked left and looked right. There were no other cars on the road. This short street seemed to be lined with houses. Some of the homes were very old, and some were newer. Some looked abandoned, while others looked lived in.

"Which way should we go?" Kate asked.

"Let's try left," Judy suggested. "I am sure we won't get lost in a village of this size."

Kate turned left. Judy had made a good choice. The second street they came to seemed to be the village's main street. An old church was on the corner. Kate made a right-hand turn.

Beside the church was a tiny post office. Next to the post office was a war memorial. Across the street, there was a community hall. There didn't seem to be anyone outside.

Kate drove a little further. She passed through a small intersection. She could see that a bit further ahead, across the next corner were train cars.

"Oh, look," Judy said, "Someone has painted sunflowers on the railcars. They look just like the statue we saw when we came into town."

At the corner before the railway, Kate noticed a little cafe. It seemed to be the only business in town. There were two cars parked in front.

"Should we pop in here?" Kate asked.

"Sounds good," said Judy.

They parked and got out. They had a stretch, then strolled inside. They were surprised when they stepped inside. The decor was white and gold. The cafe looked like it could be in Paris or Beverly Hills. They hadn't expected something so posh in such a tiny village.

A young man greeted them, "Hello," he said.

Kate noted that he was quite handsome. "Hi," she replied.

"How can I help you, ladies, on this beautiful Saturday?" he asked.

Behind a glass counter, there were cakes, pastries, and loaves of bread. There were also beverage options, including various coffees, teas, and lattes.

There was so much to choose from that neither Judy nor Kate knew what to pick. There was a decadent-looking chocolate cake. There were lemon danishes. There was baklava. Pastel-colored macarons were tempting. Six flavors of muffins made deciding difficult. But, most intoxicating was the scent of the freshly baked bread.

A grey-haired lady sat at a table in the corner. Then, sensing their indecision, she said, "You can't go wrong with any of it. Your best bet is to get one of everything."

Judy laughed, "That does sound like a solution."

In the end, Judy settled on a caramel latte with an apple muffin. She also purchased a loaf of rye bread, half a dozen oatmeal cookies, and a piece of carrot cake for later.

Kate ordered a hot chocolate and a piece of coconut cream pie. She bought a loaf of raisin bread, four butter tarts, and a slice of cheesecake to take home.

As she got her goodies, she said, "Cheesecake, my favorite."

They took their goodies to a table near the grey-haired lady. When they bit into their baked goods, they were not disappointed.
"Good, isn't it?" the lady asked.
"Mmmhmmm," Judy and Kate both nodded. This baking was amazing.
"Tyler is a real treasure," the lady said.

Kate looked back to the counter where the handsome young man had been. But, unfortunately, he was no longer there. Kate assumed he had gone backroom to do more of his baking.

"My name is Beth," the lady added. "We are very lucky to have Tyler in our little village. People come from hours away to get some of his baking. You folks are lucky it's still the spring. He'd be completely sold out in the summer months by now."

Judy and Kate introduced themselves to Beth.

"You wouldn't happen to be familiar with anyone with the last name Munro?" Kate asked.

Beth thought, "No, I don't think I am, but I have only lived in these parts for a few years."

Judy sighed. That would have been too easy, she thought. But, before she could get disappointed, she heard a voice say, "Munro? That was my mother's maiden name."

Judy and Kate both turned to see the handsome, young baker, Tyler smiling at them.

Chapter 8 Discussion Questions

1. What was the school like that you attended?

   _____
   _____
   _____

2. What did you like to play when you were a child?

   _____
   _____
   _____

3. Do you prefer coffee or tea?

   _____

4. What are your favorite kinds of sweets and baked goods?

   _____
   _____
   _____
   _____

Chapter 9

"Really?" Judy exclaimed. "You're part of the Munro family?"

"I am," said Tyler, "Though I wasn't raised around here and only know a handful of people from that side of my family. So who are you looking for?"

"Alva Munro," Judy said. "Or anyone that might know her. We don't know if she'd even still be alive."

Tyler shook his head, "I'm sorry. That name does not sound familiar."

Judy sighed.

"Can I ask why you're looking for this, Alva Munro?" Tyler asked.

Judy explained to him about finding the letter in the wooden trunk. She then pulled out the letter and showed it to Tyler.

He took the letter. He carefully studied it.

"Wow," he said. "This is truly amazing. It's still sealed."

Judy told him how she hadn't felt right about opening it. She had hoped to find Alva Munro or one of her relatives and give the letter to them.

"That is what brought us to Fox Creek today," Kate added.

Tyler was impressed. He thought for a moment. Then he said, "The letter is addressed to Mrs. Alva Munro. The stamp is from 1955. A woman that was a wife in that year would be at least in her eighties now."

Kate and Judy agreed.

"My Great-Aunt Gloria is a bit younger than that, but she still lives in the area. Her maiden name was Munro."

"Oh, that could be a good lead," Judy said as she smiled.

Tyler explained how his Great-Aunt Gloria was the reason he had moved to Fox Creek. Gloria had been his mom's dearly loved aunt. Tyler had been born and raised in Vancouver, but his parents had brought him to visit Fox Creek every few years. Gloria and her husband, Bill, had made the trip to Vancouver twice a year to see Tyler's family.

"When Uncle Bill passed away last year, I couldn't bear the thought of Aunt Gloria here on her own. I was finding my job in the city uninspiring, so I thought I would take a chance. Starting this small business in a tiny rural village has actually been good for business." Tyler added, "More importantly, it has been good for my soul."

"It hasn't been so good for my waistline," Beth chimed in. "But absolutely worth it."

"It's a great story," Judy said. "You never know folks' stories by looking at the surface. I never imagined a cafe like this on our drive here today."

"You've got a pretty interesting story too with your letter," Tyler said. "I've got a few more hours of work. I couldn't tempt you to wait around until I am done? I could take you to meet Aunt Gloria."

Judy and Kate were happy with the idea.
"I will even bring supper," Tyler added.
"Well, then you definitely have a deal," Judy laughed.

Chapter 9 Discussion Questions

1. Where was your family originally from?
   _____
   _____

2. Have you lived in different places?
   _____
   _____
   _____

3. Where was a favorite place for you to visit?
   _____
   _____

4. Do you prefer small towns, big cities or out in the country?
   _____

Chapter 10

Judy and Kate promised to be back at the cafe at 5 pm. They had decided they would go out and do a little exploring.

Judy and Kate grabbed their cameras. First, they took some pictures of the cafe. Then they decided to take photos of the train cars with sunflowers painted.

"These will be great on Instagram," Kate said.
"I don't even know what that is," replied Judy.
"We'll have to get you set up, Gram. Your photographs are always so great. You'd have a tonne of followers."
Judy wasn't sure what exactly followers were, but she figured she had gotten along fine until now without any.

Since it was a lovely day, they decided to walk up one side of the street and back down the other side. Judy wanted to go and see the old church. She was sure it was the same church as in the Fox Creek book she borrowed from the library.

"I have a great idea," she said to Kate. "I could try to get a photograph of the church at the same angle as the picture in the book."

"That would be cool," Kate agreed, "Two pictures taken over a hundred years apart of the same church."

At the old church, they learned that Sunday services still happened every week.

A robin chattered to them. They took that as a good sign.

"Hello there," Judy said to the little bird, "What are you trying to tell us?"

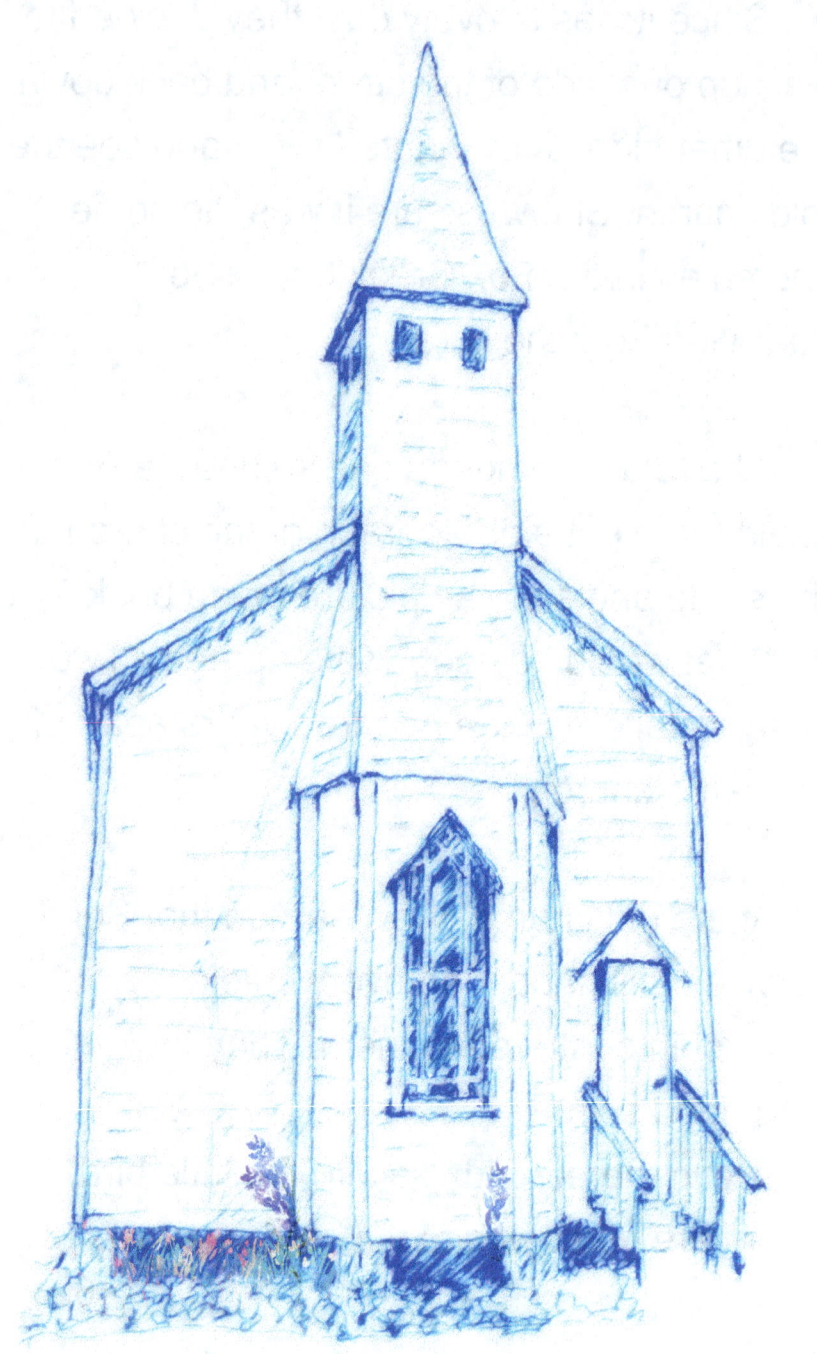

They were sure to get the robin into a couple of the pictures. Though the building was old, it had been well maintained. You could tell that the community still cared for this place.

Judy took a picture of Kate in front of the church. Then Kate showed Judy how they could take a selfie together with Kate's phone.

Judy was still laughing at this as they walked back to Kate's truck.
"Where should we go now?" Kate asked.
"We could stop at the old schoolhouse," Judy suggested. "We could get some nice pictures of that."
"Good idea," Kate agreed.
They stopped and explored the old schoolhouse for almost a half hour. Once again, they got lots of photos with their cameras.

The children had left the playground, so Kate went over and sat on one of the swings.

Judy laughed as Kate started to swing higher and higher, like a little girl.

"Should I jump?" Kate teased as she swung high.

"I don't know if I'll be much help if you break your leg," Judy warned.

"Yeah, I better not," Kate relented. She slowed her swing down. "I wouldn't want to show up to my new job with broken bones. They might regret hiring me."

Kate motioned to the swing beside her. "Have a swing, Gram," she said.

"Oh, I couldn't," Judy replied.

"Why not?"

"Well, I don't know," Judy said.

She sat down on the swing beside Kate's. She couldn't remember how long it had been since she sat on a swing. She felt a little silly, but as no one was around to see her, she started to swing. She didn't go as high as Kate, but this was fun. She was reminded of a swing her father had made and hung on the branch of the old sycamore tree by the pond. Oh, how she and her sister, Marie, used to quarrel over that swing.

Afterward, it was good to get in Kate's truck, drink cool water, and put on the air conditioning. Although it was only spring, it was getting to be quite a hot day.

Kate looked at the clock. "Well," she said, "We still have a few hours before it's five o'clock. What should we do now?"

There was not much to do in Fox Creek. Judy shrugged. She wasn't sure where they should head now.

"We could head back towards the road that brought us here. But, we could go in another direction and see what adventure we might find," Kate suggested

Judy chuckled, " Yes, I have no doubt; wherever we go, you will be able to find some sort of adventure."

Chapter 10 Discussion Questions

1. Did you/do you go to church?
   _____

2. If you went to church or Sunday school, are there songs you remember or like to sing?
   _____

3. Are you on social media such as Facebook, Instagram, or Twitter? If so, what do you enjoy about social media?
   _____

4. Did you have a brother or sister? Did you ever quarrel as children
   _____
   _____

5. What was your favorite thing to do on the playground?
   _____
   _____

Chapter 11

As they reached the road that had led them to Fox Creek, they turned in the opposite direction they had come. They only went a short distance when Kate felt compelled to turn onto another road.

"Don't get us lost," Judy warned.
"I'm looking for more moose," Kate smiled.
They approached what looked to be an old road. It didn't look like it got much traffic these days. Both women noticed an old sign that said Munro Homestead, with an arrow pointing down this dirt road.

"Oh my goodness!" Kate exclaimed. "Should we check it out?"
"I sure would like to," Judy replied.
So, the pair turned down the dirt road to see if they could find the homestead.

Since the road was dirt, Kate drove a little slower than usual. Once again, they found themselves in a spot filled with silence. There were no other cars. There were no houses or people. There were no animals to be seen.

At their slow pace, it seemed to take a long time. Finally, they saw another sign noting the homestead was two miles away.

"We're almost there," Kate said. "I wonder what it looks like."

"I hope it gives us a clue," Judy said.

Kate continued to drive at a slow speed towards a grove of trees. "It must be right past there," she pointed.

Suddenly, the dirt road turned a little muddy. Kate stepped on the gas to go a little faster and get through the mud. But unfortunately, the mud seemed to get deeper, and the truck seemed to be sinking.

"Oh no," she said, "We just have to get past this patch. We're almost there."

That is when the truck stopped moving. Kate turned the wheel. She stepped on the gas. She tried putting it in reverse. It was no use. They were stuck. Kate sighed. "I shouldn't have tried to cross through the mud, but we were so close."

Sure enough, they were pretty close to the homestead now. But, there were still trees blocking their view.

"It's all right," Judy said. "We'll figure something out."

Kate stepped out of the truck. She could now see that the mud was up the tires. It seemed to have all happened so fast. One minute they were cruising down the dirt road; the next, the truck was half buried in mud. She felt so silly.

Praying that they would have cell service out here, Kate reached into the vehicle to grab her cell phone. Judy stepped out. She saw the pickle they found themselves in. She had to laugh.

"Well," she said, "We were looking for an adventure."

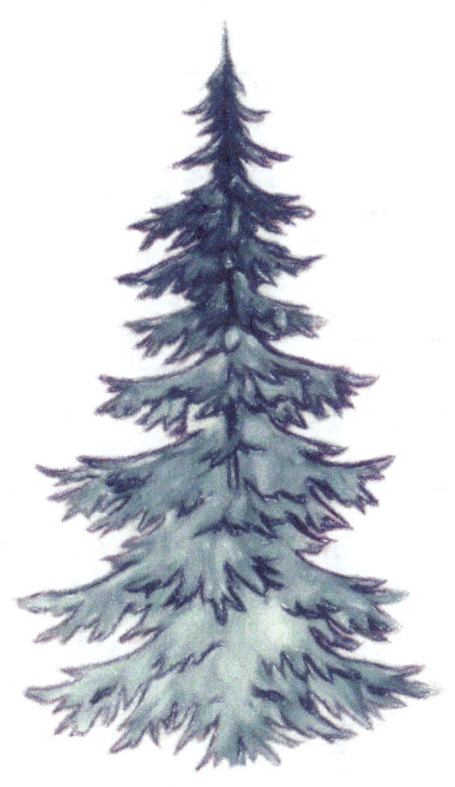

Chapter 11 Discussion Questions

1. Have you visited old homesteads or old homes?

_____

_____

2. What is your favorite kind of house?

_____

_____

3. Share a time when you had some sort of car trouble.

_____

_____

_____

4. Cell phones can be useful. Are there any times in the days before cell phones that you could have really used one?

_____

_____

_____

Chapter 12

Judy and Kate managed to get themselves to some drier ground. Kate was grateful to see that there was cell service in that location. She hadn't been sure. They seemed to be out in the middle of nowhere.

A quick search and Kate found a number for a local tow truck company. She was again thankful when someone picked up right away.

Kate explained the situation they were in and described where they were. She mentioned the Munro homestead, and the fellow on the phone seemed to know exactly where they were.

But, he said he was finishing up another job. So it might be over an hour before he made it to them.

Kate gave Judy an update. Judy shrugged. There was nothing to be done about it.

"Well," said Judy, "Should we make our way to check out that homestead?"

"Definitely," replied Kate. "After all this trouble, it sure better be worth it."

Judy was glad that she had worn comfy shoes. The ground was uneven as the pair steered clear of the mud. She was also happy that Kate remembered the water bottles as the day continued to get warmer.

The place came into view. They saw that the homestead seemed more of an estate than what they imagined as a homestead. It seemed abandoned. Yet, it looked like someone still cared for and maintained the place.

"Look at this place," Kate gushed.

Judy imagined the family that had lived there. She imagined the picture she saw of Alva Munro with her hair in victory rolls.

She imagined the small child in the picture and the love between the pair. What it must have been like to see this home filled with people.

Judy looked around the garden. Though they hadn't started to bud, she could make out old rosebushes in front of the home. She wished she could see them when they bloomed this summer.

"Isn't this place marvelous?" said Kate in awe. "Imagine living in a place like this."

Judy spotted the first butterfly of spring. She followed it up the stairs of the front porch. She couldn't resist but try the front door. It was locked. She peered in the window and saw that the place was still furnished. She noted a vase of fresh purple tulips on a wooden table. Someone had been here recently.

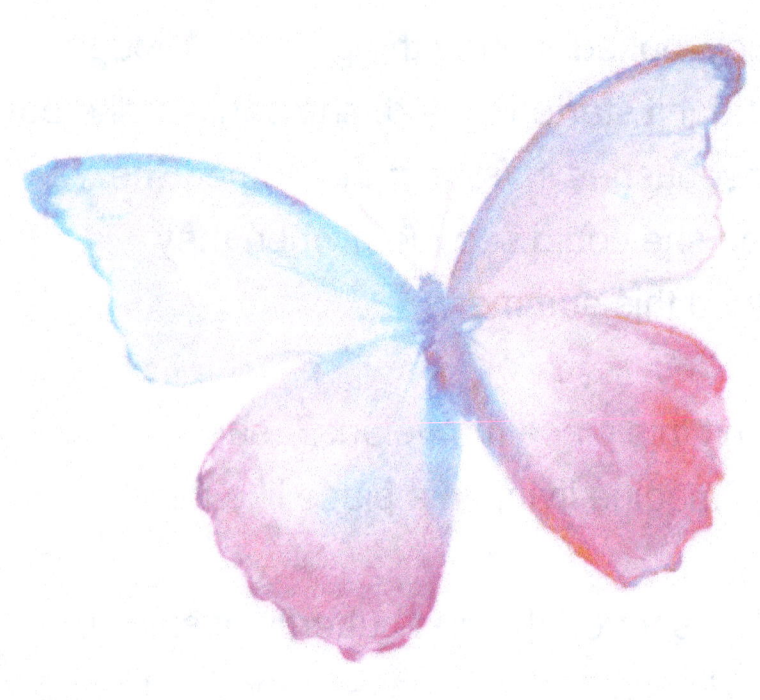

Kate was off a distance in the yard, "Look, Gram," she called out. "You've got to come to see this."

Judy crossed the yard in the direction of Kate's voice. "Where are you?" she called.

"Over here," Kate answered from behind some shrubbery. "Look, I think this is a maze!"

"This is unbelievable."

"Let's follow it and see where it takes us."

"I don't know," said Judy, but Kate's enthusiasm was contagious, and she followed her granddaughter.

There were twists and turns. Judy was sure they got lost a few times. After quite some time, they discovered the maze opened to a second road. It was older, in disrepair, but paved.

"Now, this is the road we should have taken, and we wouldn't have gotten stuck in the mud." Kate joked.

"Oh no," Judy said. "We better get back for the tow truck."

Judy and Kate had lost track of time, so they hurried back to the old Munro homestead. As they exited the maze, they were startled when a voice called out. "I imagine you are the ladies who called for a tow truck."

Judy looked up to see a handsome, grey-haired man sitting on the veranda. A flush crept over her face. Kate's eyebrows raised ever so slightly as she watched her grandmother.

Judy cleared her throat, "Yes," she answered. "We got ourselves into a bit of a mess."

"I got us into a bit of mess," Kate corrected.

"I could see that. Not from around here, I reckon, or you'd know that dirt road is not a good idea in spring." the fellow replied. "Well, no worries. We'll get you out."

"My name is Robert Clark," he added.

Judy and Kate introduced themselves, then followed Robert back to the truck. As he worked, Judy noticed that he was a strong, capable man, though a man of few words. When she saw Kate watching her, she directed her gaze to a nearby tree.

Kate looked at her watch. They were still supposed to meet Tyler. She hoped they wouldn't be late.

Thankfully, Robert knew what he was doing. In a fraction of Judy and Kate's time exploring the old Munro homestead, Robert had Kate's truck out of the mud.

"It'll need a good wash," Robert said. "I imagine the mud is everywhere. If you want to bring it back to my garage, my guys will give it a good look over."

"That's very kind of you," Kate answered. "Are you sure it's no problem? We are invited for supper in Fox Creek."

"No problem at all," he said. "Stop by the garage after supper, and it should be good to go."

Robert said they could follow him back. He would keep a good eye on them to make sure there were no issues with the truck.

While driving, Kate commented, "He sure is a silver fox, Gram."

Judy flushed again, "A what?"

"You know, an attractive older man with silver hair."

Judy looked straight ahead, "Attractive?" she asked. "I hadn't noticed."

Kate laughed. "Yeah, right, and I hadn't noticed that the guy in the cafe was attractive."

When they arrived back in Fox Creek, Robert turned right where they had turned left their first time in town. They made a left turn down three blocks and arrived at a large garage. The sign showed that Robert Clark was the local mechanic and a tow truck driver.

The yard was full of restored cars from the 1920s to the 1970s.

"Wow, this is so cool," Kate said.

"Very impressive," Judy agreed. She would have loved to have a good look at all these cars. Yet, she was also anxious to see if she could learn more about the mysterious letter.

Robert shrugged. "Just a little hobby I have in my retirement."

"I adore that green 1920s Dodge Brothers sedan," Kate said.

"You know cars and have some taste," said Robert. Then he asked Judy, "Do you have any favorites?'

She looked around. "I'd have to say that one right there," she said, pointing to a 1940s pick-up truck. There was nothing fancy about it. It hadn't been restored like some of the others. It seemed to be a mix of original paint and rust, but there was something charming about the weathered patina. The grill looked original. The truck was a survivor, still here after all these decades.

Robert smiled.

"You ladies were sure off the beaten path today," he noted.

"We sure were," Judy agreed but offered no more information about what had taken them there.

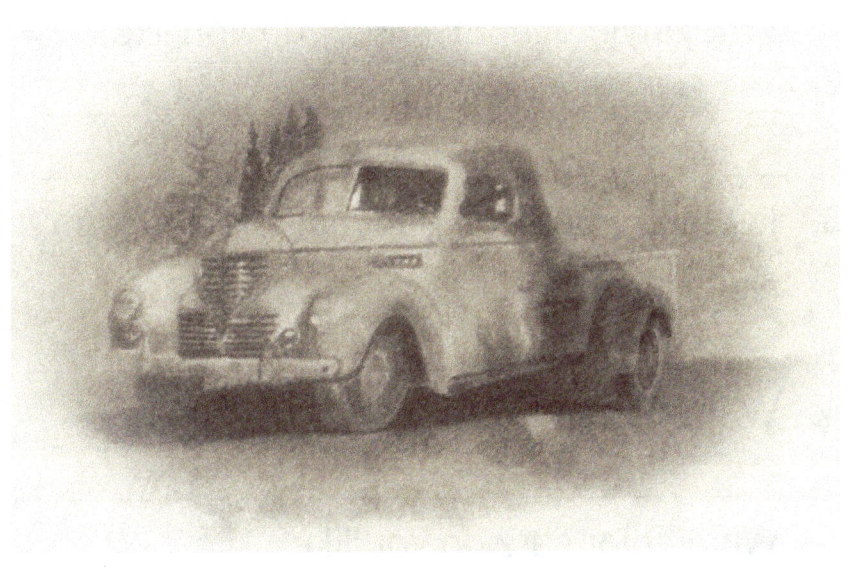

Chapter 12 Discussion Questions

1. Where are some places you have explored?
   _____
   _____

2. What style of home decor do you like?
   _____
   _____

3. Is there a particular decade of cars you like?
   _____

4. What is your favorite car?
   _____

5. What color cars do you like?
   _____

Chapter 13

Judy and Kate didn't make it back to the cafe until 5:15. Tyler had waited. He was keeping himself busy with some tidying. They told him all about their afternoon's adventure.

"Wow," he said. "I never knew about that old homestead. I will have to ask Aunt Gloria about it. I could take a drive out."

"Well, I'd suggest you wait till the ground dries up or take that alternate road," Kate suggested.

It was a short walk to Tyler's aunt's house. He had several bags carrying the supper he had promised.

He knocked before walking inside the tiny, white cottage-style home. Gloria greeted Tyler with a hug.

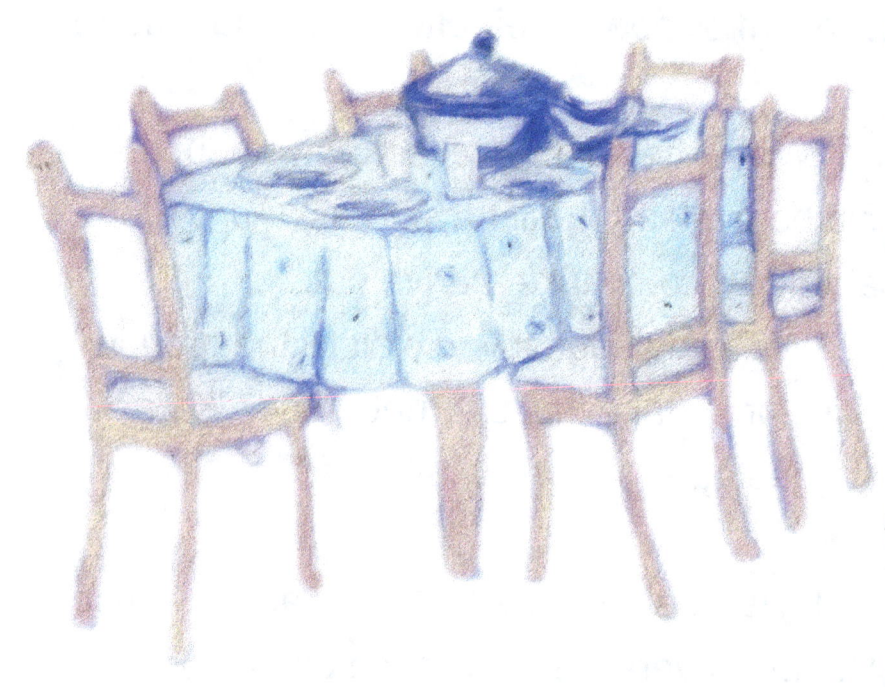

To Judy and Kate, she said, "Welcome, welcome. Tyler said he was bringing guests to dinner. Do you have a girlfriend you haven't told me about Tyler?" she asked eyeing Kate.

It was Kate's turn to blush.

"No," Tyler stammered, also blushing. "These are some nice folks that came into the cafe looking to learn more about some local history."

Gloria smiled, "Well, come on in. We'll have some food, and I will see if I can help you out."

Tyler's meal did not disappoint. Judy was eager to ask Gloria questions. But, Tyler's lasagna, Caesar salad, and garlic bread were worth the wait.

As Tyler dished out some apple caramel cheesecake for dessert, Gloria brought out a pot of tea.

"Cheesecake, my favorite," Kate smiled.

"I know," Tyler said.

Kate looked at him, and for a brief moment, their eyes locked.

"This is delicious," Gloria exclaimed.

There was silence as everyone dug into their dessert.

After Gloria cleared the dishes, she said, "So what are you ladies looking to learn about the history of Fox Creek?"

"We are looking for information about Alva Munro," said Judy, "Or the Munro family."

Gloria went still. She let out a soft sigh and dropped to her seat,

"Are you okay, Aunt Gloria," Tyler asked, reaching for her.

Gloria brushed her hand in the air, "I'm okay. I haven't heard that name in a very long time."

"So you know her?" Kate asked.

Judy shook her head, encouraging Kate to slow down.

"I knew her, yes," answered Gloria. "She was the wife of my favorite cousin."

Judy noticed how Gloria used the past tense and deduced that Alva Munro must not still be alive.

"I've never heard of her," Tyler said.

"Sad story," Gloria murmured. "But one from a very long time ago."

After a few more minutes of silence, Gloria composed herself and asked, "May I ask what this could be about? Alva has been gone a very long time."

Judy went to her purse and got the letter. She placed it in front of Gloria. "I found this in an old wooden trunk at an antique shop." Gloria brushed her fingers over the envelope. "It sure looks old. So you didn't open it?'

Judy shook her head. "I didn't feel right about it. I had to see if she was alive or had family still around. I guess the letter belongs to you."

"No," Gloria said. "The letter would belong to Robert Clark."

Kate and Judy looked at each other.
Tyler said what they both were thinking, "Robert Clark? You met him this afternoon."

Chapter 13 Discussion Questions

1. What are some of your favorite meals?
___
___
___

2. Do you like to cook?
___

3. Who was a great cook in your family? What was a recipe they're known for?
___
___
___

4. Did you have cousins or other family members you have been close with?
___
___
___
___

Chapter 14

Gloria offered no explanation of how Robert Clark was connected to Alva Munro. She got up and gave him a call.

"Robert," she said. "Could you come over? I have something here you might want to see."

Fox Creek was so small that the group didn't have to wait long before Robert arrived.

When he came in, he seemed surprised to see Judy and Kate.

"What's up?" he asked.

Gloria offered him a chair, and Tyler passed him a piece of cheesecake. Nobody could turn down Tyler's desserts.

As he ate, Gloria passed the envelope to him. Robert glanced at it. Then his eyes jumped back to the old envelope. "What's this?" he asked.

Judy explained about the old wooden trunk she had bought at the antique shop.

Robert was now holding the envelope, inspecting it. "It's never been opened."

"Are you going to open it?" Gloria asked.

"What good would it do now?" Robert replied.

Kate couldn't help her curiosity. She asked, "Did you know Alva Munro?'

"She was my mother," said Robert.

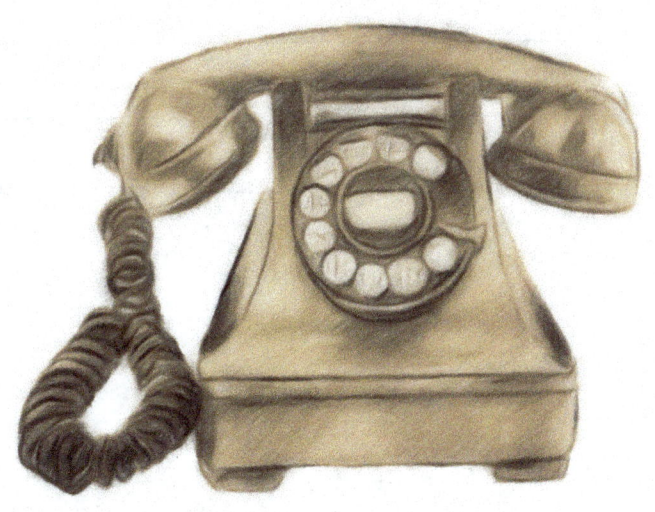

Chapter 14 Discussion Questions

1. If an old family letter turned up, would you open it?

   _____

2. Have you kept any old letters?

   _____

   _____

3. What other keepsakes have you kept?

   _____

   _____

   _____

   _____

Chapter 15

The room was tense as the group sat around the table. An awkward silence filled the space.

Robert stood up and went to the window.

"Perhaps we should be going," Judy said as she started to get up.

Gloria spoke up before she could, "You asked what good it would do now, but what harm could it do now."

"I don't know," Robert said. "It's all so long ago."

"I don't know either," Gloria said. "But something tells me you should open it. There's got to be a reason it landed in the hands of this kind woman. She went to all this trouble to return it to where it belonged. It belongs to you though, and it's for you to decide."

Robert sat back down.

Judy noticed that the man who seemed so strong and capable with Kate's truck was now unsteady. His aqua eyes were watery. She was starting to regret coming. Her intention had not been to bring up difficult memories.

Robert reached for the envelope. Then, slowly, he started to open it. As he read, a single tear slid down his cheek. When he finished, he passed the letter to Judy.

"Here," he said. "You found this. I want you to read it too."

Surprised, Judy said, "Oh, I don't know." She looked to Gloria, who nodded.

After Judy read the letter, Robert asked if she would read it to the group.

"I want everyone to know what it says, but I won't get the words out."

Judy started to protest but relented. How could she deny this request?

She cleared her throat and began.

Dearest Alva,

I am so very sorry for the trouble I have caused you. I am so ashamed of what I have done and need to confess my sins to you.

On the night of June 30th, I was out at your old place. Mr. Evans declared his love for me in the maze and gave me a sapphire ring. He made promises to me that evening, and I believed him like the silly fool I was. I snuck out through the maze in glee, thinking we'd finally be together.

I'd later learn that you had been out to the place a few days before. You had been begging Mrs. Evans for the ring your husband had proposed to you with. A sapphire ring, your birthstone.

Apparently, upon seeing a blonde woman in the maze from her bedroom window, Mrs. Evans went to the safe.

When she found the ring missing she immediately called the police. Of course, her husband could not admit his infidelity. He supported her claims that you must have stolen the sapphire ring.

You will know that when the police questioned you, a search did not produce the ring. It didn't matter though, the damage was done.

Even though it has been several months, the rumors around town persist. Your reputation has been irreparably damaged. I knew I had to do something, but I am so ashamed of my part in this mess. I would die if my parents knew I was carrying on with a married man.

I'm leaving this evening on a train to the east. I have no plans of returning to Fox Creek. I encourage you to take this letter to the police.

If they go to your old place they will find the sapphire ring. It is in a silver box buried under the rosebush on the left side of the front porch. I snuck back to the property and buried it there while the Evans family was away for Thanksgiving.

It is my hope that your name will be cleared with this letter and when the ring is found on the Munro Homestead property.

With deepest regrets

The letter was unsigned except for the letter B.

"Bonnie," said Gloria.

Everyone at the table looked at the woman.

"My big sister," she explained. "She left the autumn of 1955 and never returned."

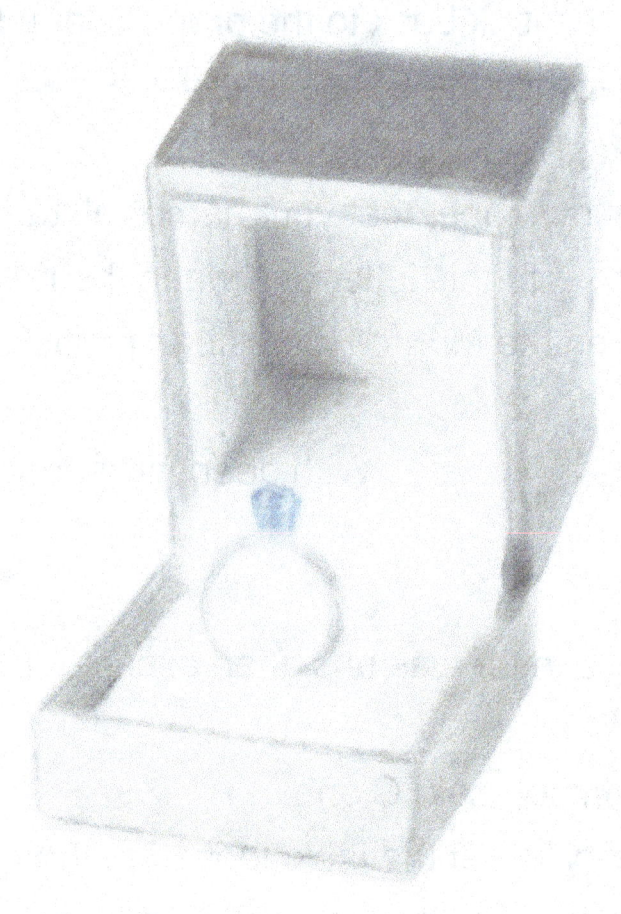

Chapter 15 Discussion Questions

1. What did you think the letter would say?
   _____
   _____
   _____

2. How would you feel if you were accused of something you didn't do?
   _____
   _____
   _____

3. Robert wants the group to know what the letter says. It is good to have support from others. Who can you turn to when you need some support?
   _____
   _____

Chapter 16

Judy felt like she and Kate were interlopers. She thought they should leave but didn't know how they could make an appropriate exit.

"Maybe I was wrong," Robert said, "Maybe it will do some good."

The group looked at him as he seemed to collect his thoughts.

"I mean, it doesn't do my mother any good, but the truth coming out could be good. I never believed she did it."

"Can I ask what happened to her?" Kate said.

"She couldn't handle the accusations," Robert said. "1955 had already been a rough year with my father passing. After he was gone, she couldn't afford the homestead. Then, she found out about some debts he had. So she lost the house and everything in it to Mr. Evans."

He continued, "We went to live with my grandparents, her parents. Things were rough enough, and then the claims that she was a thief. It was too much for her. My grandparents sent her to live with some relatives in Calgary for a while. They thought things might cool down after a while, and she could return."

"I remember it all so well," Gloria said. "Folks around here mistreated her."

"Yeah," Robert agreed. "And they never let up, even after she was gone. My childhood was not a whole lot of fun. My grandparents thought if they changed my last name to theirs' the kids would leave me alone. That didn't happen."

Gloria reached over and squeezed his hand.

"She passed away at the end of 1955."

Robert seemed to sense everyone was curious about how she died but was too polite to ask.

"My grandparents said she died of a broken heart. That's all I know," Robert offered.

Robert shared how, as soon as he turned eighteen, he left Fox Creek and left for Alberta. After some time he found work in the oil fields. He only returned years later to care for his aging grandparents.

"It's amazing that after all this time, you found the letter, Judy," said Tyler.

"How did you say you found it?" Robert asked.

Judy repeated the story of their trip to the antique shop and how she had discovered the letter in a wooden trunk."

"I sure would love to see that wooden trunk," said Robert.

"I have a picture of it on my phone," offered Kate. She went to Robert's side, scrolled through her many photos, and brought up a picture of the trunk to show him.

"Well, I'll be," he said. "That trunk was in grandpa's den for as long as I can remember. That letter was right there my whole childhood."

"It must have come after Alva left," Gloria suggested. "Then, it was either forgotten about after she died, or your grandpa didn't see the point of opening it."

Robert looked at Judy. "I don't know the reason why that letter surfaced after all these years, but there must be one. So I do thank you for going to all this trouble to return it."

"So," asked Kate, "Are we going to go and see if the sapphire ring is still there?"

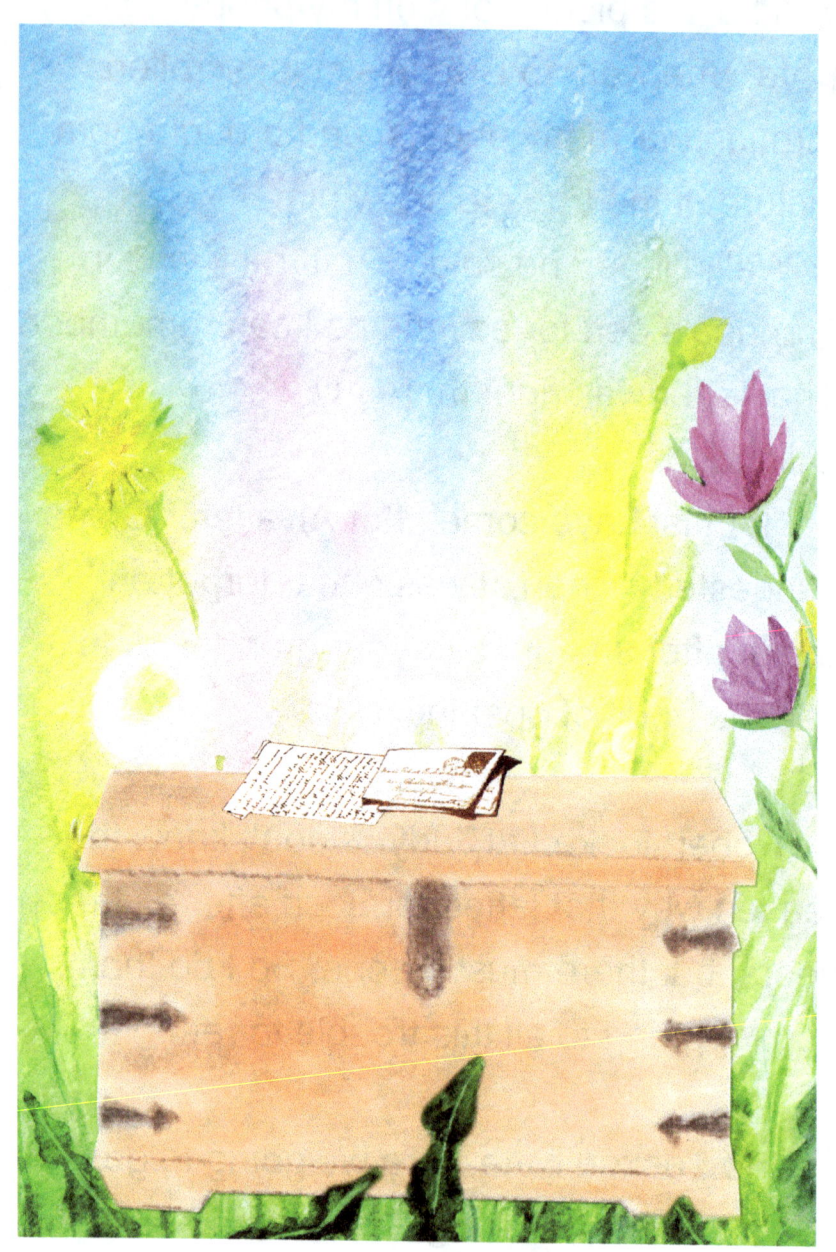

Chapter 16 Discussion Questions

1. Did you live your whole life in your hometown? Or did you leave your hometown?
   _____

2. If you left your hometown, where did you go? Do you ever visit or miss your hometown?
   _____
   _____

3. If you stayed in your hometown your whole life, is there anywhere you ever thought about moving to?
   _____
   _____

4. What is your favorite gemstone?
   _____

5. What is your birthstone?
   _____

Chapter 17

"Do you know who owns the old Munro Homestead," Judy asked, "They might not like us digging up their rosebushes."

"I own it," Robert said with a smile. "Let's do it!"

"You bought your family's old home," Tyler asked.

"Yeah," said Robert. "1955 was a terrible year. Of course, the years after weren't so great either. Those early years of my life though, they were the best."

The group returned to Robert's garage and piled in Kate's truck. Robert shared memories of happy times with his mother and father in the old Munro Homestead. He told how with money he had saved from working, he was able to buy the place when it came up for sale.

"Turn here," he advised Kate. "We don't want to take the dirt road. The tow truck driver will do you no good if you got stuck again."

Kate took the alternate road to the place. Then Robert led them through the maze to the property.

Tyler offered to dig, but Robert said, "No, I've got to do this."

It took less than 10 minutes. Robert picked up the silver box, and after almost seventy years, Alva Munro's name was finally cleared.

Afterward—4 Months Later

Judy handed Kate her bouquet. "You look beautiful," she said.

"Thank you, Gram," replied Kate. "I love your plaid dress."

Judy had picked a beige plaid dress special for Kate.

Kate had returned to the antique shop and purchased the soft pink Victorian dress she had eyed in the spring.

"You were right that day at the antique shop. There were reasons you were meant to get that old wooden trunk. For one thing, I would never have met Tyler if you hadn't."

Judy was happy to see how her granddaughter's life was unfolding. She was blossoming into such a wonderful woman.

"We should sneak out and take a selfie in front of the church like we did our first time in Fox Creek," Kate suggested.

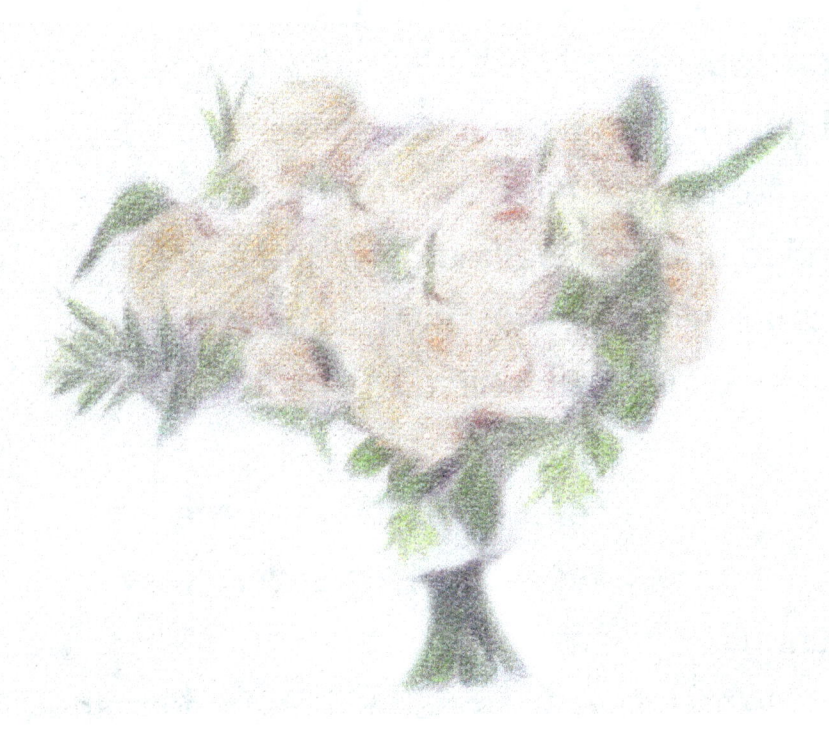

"You can't let the groom see you before the wedding," cautioned Judy.

Kate laughed as she grabbed her grandmother's hand, "We'll be stealthy."

They did make it out for their selfie with no one but their old robin friend, who was now a busy mother, none the wiser.

To Judy's relief, the groom didn't see the bride until she walked down the aisle. The small, simple ceremony was beautiful and went off without a hitch.

After the ceremony, the newlyweds chatted with the well-wishers while leaving the church.

When Kate approached her grandmother, she whispered, "Robert looks particularly handsome today. You should ask him to dance at the reception."

Judy smiled.

As the bride and groom reached the street, the 1920s green Dodge Brothers sedan awaited them. Robert was there holding the door open for the bride.

"Your chariot awaits," he teased.

When the couple drove away, Robert approached Judy.

"And for you, I brought the old truck out," he said

Being the gentleman he was, he opened the passenger door for her before getting in the driver's side.

"Are you sure it's safe," she asked.

"The truck? Of course," he replied.

"No," she said, "Driving way out to the Munro homestead."

"No mud this time of year. We'll be good."

"It will be a beautiful spot for the reception," Judy mused. "And for the wedding photos. I'm amazed that you have cared for it all these years."

"Wait till you see the roses," said Robert.

"Roses?" Judy questioned, "This late in the year?"

"My good lady, there are roses at the Munro homestead from late May until the fall."

Judy remembered seeing the barren rosebushes that spring day with Kate. She had never imagined then what life would be like now.

She took a quick glance at the man driving. Kate was right; he did look particularly handsome today. A silver fox—is that what Kate had called him? She found herself hoping that he might ask her for a dance later. Maybe, just maybe, if he didn't ask her, Judy would ask him. Judy smiled.

"A penny for your thoughts," Robert said.

"Oh, it will take a whole lot more than a penny," Judy laughed.

Discussion Questions

1. Were you surprised that Kate and Tyler got married?
   _____

2. Share some memories of a wedding that you have been to.
   _____
   _____
   _____

3. Do you like to dance?
   _____

4. What is your favorite music for dancing?
   _____

5. In your imagination, what will life bring for Kate and Tyler?
   _____
   _____
   _____
   _____

6. Do Judy and Robert dance? If so, who is the one who asked for a dance?
   _____

7. In your imagination, is there something more for Judy and Robert in the future?
   _____
   _____
   _____
   _____
   _____
   _____